HIV in Pregnancy

Prevention of Mother to Child Transmission of HIV

By

Annah Morris

Table of Contents

- <u>Medical Treatment During Pregnancy</u>

- <u>Antiretroviral Therapy</u>

- <u>Care During Labour and Delivery</u>

- <u>Postpartum Care</u>

Acronyms

ADCC	Antibody-dependent cellular cytotoxicity
ART	Antiretroviral treatment
CD4+	Cluster designation 4 positive lymphocytes
CPT	Cotrimoxazole preventive therapy
DNA	Deoxyribonucleic acid
EID	Early infant diagnosis of HIV
HIV	Human Immunodeficiency Virus
IgA	Immunoglobulin A
IgM	Immunoglobulin M
MTC	Mother-to-child
MTCT	Mother-to-child transmission
PCR	Polymerase Chain Reaction
RNA	Ribonucleic acid
SLPI	Secretory leukocyte protease inhibitor
STD	Sexually transmitted disease(s)
ZDV	Zidovudine

INTRODUCTION

HIV (the Human Immunodeficiency Infection) destroys the body's defense against different diseases, which lead to death in the event that the individual isn't dealt with fittingly with hostile to HIV drugs. HIV is transmitted through an infected person's blood and can also be found in their genital tract. It can be passed from one person to another through infected blood transfer or unprotected sex (sex without a condom). Additionally, the virus can be passed from mother to child during pregnancy, childbirth, and breastfeeding. The most common cause of HIV infection in children is mother-to-child transmission (MTCT). A number of factors contribute to the risk of MTCT, including the presence of chorioamnionitis at delivery, decreased maternal CD4 lymphocyte counts, increased maternal HIV-1 titer, and decreased maternal HIV p24 antibody level. High viral load, on the other hand, is the only independent risk factor. It is important for you to counsel pregnant women about prevention of mother-to-child transmission (PMTCT) of HIV and to test them for HIV as a routine part of antenatal care. In some developing nations, HIV infection during pregnancy is now the most common pregnancy complication. The management of pregnancy and birth is greatly impacted by this. Nearly 600,000 children will be infected by mother-to-child transmission each year, with an estimated one and a half million HIV-positive women becoming pregnant each year ,over 1600 per day. Numerous responsibilities are assigned to maternity services in HIV-endemic regions. First, to make it possible for women to be tested and to use the results to best maintain their health; second, to use the right strategies to lower the rate of HIV transmission from mother to child (MTC); thirdly, to train staff and provide equipment to prevent HIV and other pathogens from being passed from one room to another.

CHAPTER ONE

Women's Vulnerability to HIV

Infection

There are a number of biological and sociological factors why HIV-infected women in developing countries are more likely than their male counterparts to become infected.

Biological Factors

The pace of transmission of HIV from male to female is a few higher than that from female to male. It has been hypothesized that some HIV serotypes may have a higher affinity for the Langerhans cells in the cervix, making them more effective in heterosexual transmission. These cells may serve as a gateway for HIV. Inflammation or ulceration of the vagina and vulva may make it easier for the virus to get in.In many African nations, sexually transmitted diseases (STDs) are prevalent, and HIV prevalence is also high.HIV infection, as well as chlamydia infections and other sexually transmitted diseases, may be facilitated in part by inadequate treatment or "silent" diseases.

Socio-Cultural Factors

The conditions in cultures and communities that deny women control over their bodies make them more vulnerable. Women carry the dual burden of infection and caring for infected family members, and they are frequently erroneously blamed as the source of HIV infection. Many women are forced into commercial sex work in order to survive because of gender inequalities, poverty, a lack of access to education, and job opportunities. These women are very likely to get HIV. On the other hand, a lot more women are monogamous, but their safety is greatly compromised by the sexual conduct of their male partners. Women's risk of HIV infection may rise as a result of traditional practices and customs like "dry sex," female circumcision, vaginal douching with non-antiseptic compounds, and "widow cleansing."Cultural norms and pressures frequently prevent women from taking the necessary precautions to prevent infection, despite their high risk. Numerous developing nations have low rates of male condom usage. It is challenging for women to engage in protected sex because of the desire and social pressure to reproduce. In developing nations, infections are most prevalent among young women, many of whom are just beginning their reproductive lives. The majority of women will not alter their reproductive choices after receiving an HIV diagnosis. With the possible exception of the female condom, there are no methods that women can use to prevent HIV transmission without a male partner. female barrier methods remain either expensive or unavailable in the majority of developing nations, where male resistance to condom use is prevalent.

CHAPTER TWO

Effect of HIV Infection on Pregnancy

In the developed world, it has been reported that HIV infection has little effect on pregnancy outcomes or complications. It is frequently hard to decide the general commitment of HIV contamination, drug use and lacking antenatal consideration to unfriendly results in these women HIV could be a sign or direct cause of a complicated interaction between related medical and social conditions that affect pregnancy. Women who are HIV-positive have been found to have higher rates of ectopic pregnancies than women who are not infected, which suggests that the effects of other concurrent sexually transmitted diseases may be to blame. It has been reported that HIV-positive women have a higher prevalence of genital tract infections such as Neisseria gonorrhoeae, Chlamydia trachomatis, Candida albicans, and Trichomonas vaginalis. During pregnancy, HIV-positive women are more likely to get bacterial pneumonia, urinary tract infections, and other infections. In addition to these infections and parasitic infestations, pregnant women can get any HIV-related opportunistic infection. In the developing world, tuberculosis is the most prevalent opportunistic infection associated with HIV, and its diagnosis in pregnant HIV-positive women requires special attention.Herpes zoster is a common infection in young HIV-positive women, but it is uncommon in this age group if HIV is not present. HIV-positive women may have rates of preterm labor that are as high as double those of uninfected women. Membranes that rupture before birth may also be more likely in HIV-positive women, and it has been said that abruptio placentae are more common in HIV-positive women. The infants born to HIV-positive mothers have comparable birth weights. It has been reported that stillbirth rates have increased, particularly in regions where the epidemic has been present for a considerable amount of time. Asymptomatic women appear to have a lower risk, but stillbirth rates are more than double those of HIV-negative mothers. HIV-positive women also have a higher rate of infectious complications after childbirth. In women with low CD4+ counts, Cesarean sections are especially linked to higher infectious morbidity.

CHAPTER THREE

Mother-To-Child Transmission

HIV-1 can be transmitted during pregnancy, during labor, or after birth through breastfeeding.For the purpose of developing potential interventions, it is essential to have knowledge of the probable timing of transmission. It is thought that the fetus is exposed to the virus in cervico-vaginal secretions. Additionally, the method of delivery may affect the rate of transmission. It has been demonstrated that elective or emergency Cesarean sections reduce transmission, whereas membrane ruptures lasting longer than four hours increase transmission risk. At the time of birth, about half of the infected babies will have negative viral tests. Both the cell-free and cellular components of breast milk have been found to contain HIV. Although the exact contribution of each of these routes to overall transmission has not been quantified, it appears that in-utero transmission is less frequent and that a substantial proportion of infection occurs at the time of delivery or late in pregnancy. Based on the time of infant HIV detection, a working definition has been proposed for the classification of transmission timing. An infant is considered to have been infected in utero if the virus is found within 48 hours of birth. However, if viral tests are negative during the first week of life but become positive between 7 and 90 days later, an intrapartum infection is assumed.

CHAPTER FOUR

Factors Affecting Mother-to-Child Transmission of HIV

There are a number of factors that influence HIV transmission from mother to child, but not all of them are fully understood. There are viral, maternal, obstetrical, fetal, and infant factors to consider.

Viral Factors

- **Viral load**

High maternal viraemia increases the likelihood of transmission. The presence of high levels of p24 antigenemia lends credence to clinical observations of increased transmission in these circumstances, such as in advanced disease and at the time of seroconversion. An association has been demonstrated between the maternal viral load and the risk of transmission from mother to child with the development of new methods for measuring the virus, such as quantitative polymerase chain reaction (PCR) DNA and RNA. More than half of women who had viral loads of more than 50.000 RNA copies per ml at the time of delivery were found to transmit the virus. It's possible that the local viral load in cervico-vaginal secretions and breast milk is a significant factor in determining the risk of transmission during pregnancy and breastfeeding.

Viral shedding may be affected by the local immune response, vitamin A deficiency, and the presence of sexually transmitted diseases or other causes of inflammation. Although zidovudine has been shown to reduce transmission at all levels of maternal viral load, maternal antiretroviral therapy during pregnancy is thought to reduce transmission partly through the reduction of viral load. However, the mechanism may also include post-exposure prophylaxis in the child after birth. Due to the greater reductions in viral load, combination antiretroviral therapy may be more effective at preventing transmission.

Maternal Factors

- **Maternal Immunological Status**

A decreased immune status in the mother, as indicated by low CD4+ counts, low CD4+ percentages, or high CD4+/CD8 ratios, increases the likelihood of transmission to the child. Despite the possibility of an interaction between viral load and immune response, these, in turn, may be indicators of higher viral loads rather than risk factors in and of themselves. Autologous neutralizing antibody levels may be lower in women who transmit in utero compared to those who do not or who transmit intra-partum. Both antibody-dependent cellular cytotoxicity (ADCC) antibodies and antibodies to the V3 loop of the HIV-1 envelope gp120 have not been shown to be protective. IgM and IgA deficiency in breast milk has been linked to infection during breastfeeding.

- **Maternal nutritional factors**

HIV-1-positive mothers' serum vitamin A levels have been linked to the possibility of transmission. Compared to mothers who did not transmit the virus to their children, those mothers had significantly lower mean vitamin A levels. The mechanism of the vitamin A effect is unknown, but the vitamin's influence on the integrity of the vaginal mucosa or placenta and its immune stimulatory properties have been suggested. Women with vitamin A levels below 1.4 umol/l had a 4.4-fold increased risk of transmission.On the other hand, low levels of vitamin A may serve as a sign of other deficiencies or behavioral factors that influence transmission. Zinc and selenium are two other micronutrients that have been suggested to play a possible role.

Behavioral Factor

An increased rate of transmission from mother to child has been linked to a number of behavioral factors.Smoking cigarettes and taking hard drugs by mothers are two examples. Sexual activity during pregnancy that is not protected has been linked to an increased risk of transmission from mother to child.When compared to women who had protected intercourse, those who had more episodes of unprotected sex during pregnancy had a 30% transmission rate. The effect of cervical or vaginal inflammation or abrasions or an increased concentration or diversity of HIV-1 strains could be the cause of this. It has been demonstrated that STDs increase viral shedding in cervico-vaginal secretions, and there is a correlation between the presence of STDs and an increased risk of transmission during pregnancy.

Placental Factors

The virus has been linked to factors in the placenta in the process of transmission from mother to child. There have been reports of HIV-1 infection in the placenta, and since Hofbauer cells and possibly trophoblasts express CD4+, they are susceptible to infection. Early on in the epidemic, a connection was made between chorioamnionitis and increased transmission. Other placental contaminations and non-irresistible circumstances, for example, abruptio placentae have likewise been involved. Breaks in the surface of the placenta can occur at any stage of pregnancy and may be linked to transmission; however, the significance of these breaks may depend on the viral load of the mother. This effect may be caused by placental disruption as a result of smoking and drug use, which are both linked to increased transmission. Pregnancy infection of the placenta is common in areas with a high malaria prevalence.

Obstetric Factors

Obstetric factors are important determinants of transmission because the majority of mother-to-child transmission occurs during labor and delivery. Direct skin and mucous membrane contact between the infant and the mother's cervico-vaginal secretions during labor, virus ingestion from these secretions, and ascending infection to the amniotic fluid are suggested mechanisms for HIV-1 intrapartum transmission. During pregnancy, the prevalence of HIV-1 in cervico-vaginal secretions may increase by fourfold.Other possibilities include the use of fetal scalp electrodes, an episiotomy, vaginal tears, and surgical delivery. It would appear that the duration of membrane rupture is more important than the duration of labor . A major risk factor is prolonged membrane rupture, which has been linked to an increased risk of transmission. It has been demonstrated that cesarean sections protect

Fetal Factors

Transmission may be influenced by fetal genetic factors. The role of genetic factors like the CCR-5 delta32 deletion and HLA compatibility between mother and child in determining transmission risk is still poorly understood. Preterm births are more common in women with low CD4+ counts. Co-infection with other pathogens, fetal nutrition, and fetal immune status are examples of additional fetal factors

Infant Factors

In developing nations, where breast milk accounts for 30% or more of perinatal HIV infections, breastfeeding is a major factor in mother-to-child transmission. In the developed world, where the majority of HIV-positive women refuse to breastfeed, this is less common. The amount of cell-associated and free viruses in breast milk may be related to the mother's immune suppression and vitamin A level. Mucins, HIV antibodies, lactoferrin, and the secretory leukocyte protease inhibitor (SLPI) are among the other protective factors found in breast milk. Other factors, such as the mother's disease stage, breast abscesses, mastitis, nipple cracks, maternal vitamin A status, and the child's oral thrush, may also influence the risk of breast milk transmission. Other factors in the newborn may also be associated with the risks of postnatal transmission. After ingesting the virus during pregnancy or shortly before birth, HIV can enter the body via the gastrointestinal system. In the newborn gastro-intestinal tract, there is less acidity, less mucus, less IgA activity, and thinner mucosa, all of which may make transmission easier.Additionally, the immune system of the newborn may lack macrophages and T cells, making it more susceptible to infection. A post-exposure prophylaxis effect after birth appears to account for at least some of the effect of antiretroviral medications during pregnancy.

CHAPTER FIVE

Prevention of Mother to Child Transmission of HIV

All pregnant women must have access to HIV counseling and testing during the antenatal period

(HTC). Cotrimoxazole Preventive Therapy (CPT), A RV drugs, and screening for eligibility for lifelong ARV treatment are all necessities for HIV-positive women.Safe obstetrical practices, the judicious use of Cesarean sections when possible, and the provision of intra- and immediate postpartum doses of antiretrovirals to mothers and newborns are crucial steps in preventing MTCT during labor and delivery. During the postpartum period, it is essential to ensure the following:

1. Appropriate immunization for HIV-infected infants based on HIV status

2. Counseling and support for infant feeding

3. Monitoring of opportunistic infections and the provision of CPT

4. The appropriate ARV to prevent MTCT during the breastfeeding period

5. EID of HIV infection

6. The provision of ART for HIV-infected infants who have been confirmed to be infected.

The following steps are included in the postpartum regimen for mothers:

1. ongoing HIV care and treatment, including antiretrovirals (ARVs) (lifetime ART or prophylaxis as needed)

2. The treatment and prevention of opportunistic

infections, such as tuberculosis

3. Providing comprehensive treatment and care,

including services for family planning.

CHAPTER SIX

Appropriate Interventions to Reduce Mother-to-Child Transmission

An intervention that is widely applicable in resource-poor settings would be ideal for reducing mother-to-child transmission. All pregnant women would be eligible for vaginal disinfection and vitamin A administration without the need for HIV positive women to be identified.

- Access to and use of appropriate antenatal, intrapartum, and postpartum care provided by adequately trained health professionals

- Adequate pre- and post-test counseling services

- The ability to pay for reliable HIV testing

- Appropriate laboratory facilities to monitor blood parameters during therapy;

- Delivery units with access to disinfectants, gloves, and clean needles;

- HIV-infected women's acceptance and uptake of the intervention;

- A Schedule that is logistically feasible to implement:in terms of dosing times and routes,

- Drug storage, and distribution

- A plan that the health service can afford.

The current antenatal and obstetric services face a number of obstacles as a result of the widespread implementation of strategies to prevent HIV transmission from mother to child. In environments with the fewest resources, such strategies are most needed.Interventions to prevent MTCT of HIV should not make existing services more difficult to use. Antenatal care services may not be of sufficient quality to support these interventions because they are not widely available, accessible, or utilized in many areas. These administrations should be reinforced in the years ahead to really convey MTCT anticipation systems.Additionally, the effectiveness of any interventions that are implemented into clinical practice to reduce the risk of mother-to-child transmission outside of the context of a randomized controlled trial ought to be monitored.In order to determine whether the findings of clinical trials can be applied to the real world, it will be necessary to carefully monitor the mothers and infants of these programs. The treatment of HIV and AIDS is rapidly evolving. New drugs are made available, and they are quickly put into use in clinical settings without being thoroughly evaluated for their effectiveness. The situation is not much different during pregnancy

Immune Therapy

Alternative strategies for preventing mother-to-child transmission of HIV include active vaccination with HIV vaccines and passive vaccination with hyperimmune HIV immunoglobulin (HIVIG). Through the passive transfer of antibodies, active immunization could possibly produce immunity in both the mother and the fetus. Despite the fact that numerous Phase I/II trials are currently underway, effective vaccines have not yet been identified.

Nutritional Interventions

Following the discovery that mothers whose serum vitamin A levels were low were more likely to pass HIV to their children. Vitamin A supplementation has been suggested as a treatment for prevention. The low cost, the possibility of additional nutritional and health benefits for the mother, and the fact that the intervention could be carried out without the need for HIV testing are all potential benefits of micronutrient supplementation. Vitamin A deficiency has also been linked to higher viral loads in breast milk, and breastfeeding mothers would benefit from any reduction after supplementation. It has also been suggested that other micronutrients like zinc and selenium could be used to prevent disease.

Mode of Delivery

Cesarean segment conveyance has been related with a decrease in transmission. After taking into account factors such as maternal disease stage, birth weight, antiretroviral therapy, and elective cesarean section, the risk of MTCT was reduced by more than 50% with elective cesarean section in some centers.The possibility of maternal morbidity and mortality, the availability of safe operating facilities, the potential for increased service commitments, and the accessibility of maternity services for women with subsequent pregnancies must all be taken into consideration when using cesarean sections.

Vaginal Cleansing

It has been hypothesized that, in order to cut down on HIV-1 transmission during labor and delivery, antiseptic or antiviral medications could be used to clean the birth canal. Scandinavian studies demonstrated that chlorhexidine lavage can reduce the transmission of group B streptococci. The idea is appealing for HIV prevention because it would be a low-cost intervention that could be carried out in the majority of health care settings, would not require the identification of HIV-positive women prior to the intervention, and could have additional benefits for health. Benzalkonium chloride has been proposed as an alternative antiseptic for vaginal lavage. The antiseptic should be used at 36 weeks of pregnancy to get the most benefit. In situations where resources are limited, the intervention of vaginal cleansing remains a viable option.

Modification of Infant Feeding Practice

In developing nations, where one in seven children born to HIV-positive mothers will be infected through breast milk, breastfeeding accounts for a significant portion of mother-to-child transmission. The debate regarding the appropriate feeding of infants has almost exclusively focused on the risks and benefits of breastfeeding for the infant. Breastfeeding may double the transmission rate and may be the primary factor determining the difference in transmission rates between developed and developing nations. Other potential modifications of infant feeding practices include complete avoidance of breastfeeding, early weaning, pasteurization of breast milk, and avoiding breastfeeding in the presence of breast abscesses or cracked nipples. The potential effects of breastfeeding and the resulting weight loss on the mother's immunity and long-term prognosis are among the concerns regarding the effect of breastfeeding on maternal health in HIV-positive women. The function of immunologically active components in breast milk from severely immune suppressed or malnourished mothers as well as the effects of advanced disease or nutritional deficiencies on the risk of transmission in breast milk must also be taken into consideration. If it were possible to identify infants who were already infected with HIV when they were born, breast milk might be beneficial. The advantages and disadvantages of breastfeeding in relation to HIV infection should be made clear to mothers, and they should be encouraged to make an educated choice about feeding their children. They ought to receive support in making their choice. Methods tailored to the particular circumstances of HIV-positive mothers must be promoted as alternatives to breastfeeding.

CHAPTER SEVEN

Voluntary HIV Counseling and Testing in Pregnancy

Testing of Antenatal Women

The focus has shifted from the potential public health benefits of pregnancy testing to the potential benefits for each individual woman as HIV and mother-to-child transmission knowledge has grown. This has reaffirmed the significance of providing suitable testing and counseling facilities. It is advised that pregnant women undergo testing on their own. The presentation of testing programs has expanded the quantity of distinguished HIV positive ladies in many focuses. Despite this, it may not be possible to accurately identify infected women if they do not receive antenatal care or if there are insufficient counseling and testing services.In areas of moderate or high prevalence, voluntary counseling and testing should be made available to all pregnant women who request them whenever possible. However, it is an unacceptable practice to conduct routine HIV testing on pregnant women without their consent or access to counseling. The disadvantages of doing so may negate any benefit of knowing the women's HIV status. These include stigmatization, denial of a positive diagnosis, and a reluctance to use maternity services out of fear of discrimination. However, there are a few potential advantages for pregnant women of undergoing voluntary HIV testing prior to or during pregnancy. Among these advantages are:

1. If a woman is found to be infected, this information can make it easier to get treatment and counseling right away.

2. A mother's diagnosis enables her child to receive the appropriate treatment and follow-up.

3. The woman is able to make decisions regarding her future fertility and the continuation of her pregnancy when she is aware of her HIV status.

4. The opportunity to try to prevent transmission to the child is made available by testing.

5. The woman is able to take measures to help prevent HIV transmission to sexual partners because she is aware of her HIV status.

6. Women who have been diagnosed with HIV can tell their sexual partners and allow them to get tested and counseled.

7. Women can be instructed on appropriate HIV prevention measures and risk-reduction behaviors if the test results are negative.

CHAPTER EIGHT

Management of HIV- Positive Pregnant Women

Counseling and social support are part of the multifaceted approach to HIV-positive pregnant women's medical and obstetrical care. The woman's social and mental worries might be as need might arise for clinical consideration. In all cases, pregnancy management, including antiretroviral treatment, should be viewed as only one component of the continuum of care for the mother and child. The ideal team approach would involve health professionals, counselors, and support groups. Depending on the patient's requirements and the facilities that are available, ongoing care can be provided at home, in the primary health care services, in hospitals, or in specialist clinics. The following discussion focuses on some of the management challenges faced by pregnant women who are HIV positive.

Antenatal Care

The majority of HIV-positive women will not experience any symptoms during pregnancy and will not experience any major obstetrical issues. Unless a specific HIV-related treatment is required, they should receive the same obstetric antenatal care as HIV-negative women. As an essential component of management, the HIV-positive pregnant woman's care should include ongoing counseling and support. It is necessary to provide information regarding the potential dangers of unprotected pregnancy sexual activity.

Obstetrical Management

The risk of a negative perinatal outcome for HIV-positive pregnant women will determine their antenatal care. Pregnancy care will need to be tailored to each woman, and this will be partially mitigated by other risk factors like drug use. Either regular symphesis fundal height measurements or, where available, serial ultrasound assessments can be used to evaluate fetal growth.Due to the potential for fetal infection, invasive diagnostic procedures like cordocentesis, amniocentesis, and chorion villus sampling should be avoided whenever possible. An external cephalic version of a breech fetus may result in maternal-fetal circulation leaks, so the procedure's benefits and drawbacks should be carefully considered.

Examination and Investigations

At their first visit, HIV-positive women should receive a comprehensive physical examination.Specific consideration ought to be paid to any indications of HIV-related diseases (particularly tuberculosis), oral or vaginal thrush, or lymphadenopathy. When a young woman develops herpes zoster, or shingles, it is frequently an early sign of HIV infection, and current herpes lesions or scars from an earlier infection may be visible. Other co-occurring sexually transmitted diseases, particularly syphilis, are prevalent in HIV-positive women and may raise the virus level in vaginal and cervical secretions as well as the risk of transmission. Clinical finding and treatment of vaginal or cervical irritation, unusual release or sexually transmitted disease ought to be fundamentally important. Pregnant women should be checked for signs of HIV-related opportunistic infections as well as any other concurrent infections, like infections in the urinary tract or respiratory tract. Monitor the mother's weight and, if necessary, suggest nutritional supplements. At each visit, the oro-pharynx should be checked for signs of thrush.The health service's resources will play a role in laboratory investigations.Syphilis testing ought to be embraced, and rehash testing in late pregnancy might be prudent. A complete blood count,

Haemoglobin estimation, and T cell subset investigations should be carried out whenever possible.Iron deficiency is more normal in HIV-contaminated ladies and rehashed hemoglobin tests might be useful. When available, viral load estimation may be a useful prognostic indicator.If a cervical smear has not been performed recently, it should be done. Colposcopy should only be performed on women who have abnormal results from their cervical smears.

Medical Treatment During Pregnancy

HIV-positive women should receive medical care that is tailored to their specific requirements.Although the risk to the fetus should always be considered and treatment modified if necessary, the value of vitamin A supplementation in reducing transmission has not been proven, but multivitamins may provide cost-effective nutritional support. In general, pregnancy is not a contraindication for the most appropriate antiretroviral therapy for a woman or for most of the medical management of HIV-related conditions. In areas with a high prevalence of hookworm, mebendazole should be administered at the initial visit. Pregnancy-associated malaria increases the likelihood of HIV transmission from mother to child and is associated with high rates of maternal and infant morbidity and mortality.In highly endemic areas, it is currently recommended that all primigravidae and secundigravida receive intermittent treatment with an effective, preferably one-dose antimalarial drug. This should begin in the second trimester and be administered every one to two months. Pregnancy should be treated for opportunistic infections in accordance with local policy and the clinical stage of the HIV infection. Streptomycin and pyrazinamide should not be used during pregnancy, but tuberculosis prevention and treatment should be given when necessary. Pneumocystis carinii pneumonia (PCP) prophylaxis ought to go on through pregnancy. Pentamidine or sulfamethoxazole/trimethoprim (Bactrim/ Septran) can be utilized. PCP and kernicterus have not been reported when the drug was not also used during the neonatal period. The risk to the fetus from maternal sulphonamide administration in the third trimester is outweighed by the risk to the mother's health. Pneumococcal and Hepatitis B vaccinations merit consideration. Depending on the patient's clinical stage, if treatment for opportunistic infections is required, it should be administered during pregnancy. Local policy should be followed when designing treatment plans. Additionally, when there are a variety of treatment options, the ones with the lowest fetal risk should be utilized. HIV-positive men and women frequently suffer from dermatological conditions that may necessitate prolonged treatment. After the first trimester, acyclovir can be used safely. Anti fungals with imidazole or gentian violet applied topically can be used throughout pregnancy, and oral fluconazole can be taken after the first trimester if necessary.

Antiretroviral Therapy

Antiretroviral medication during pregnancy should be considered for two reasons:the mother's health and transmission prevention. If antiretroviral therapy is prescribed for the mother, pregnancy should not be a contraindication. Adult antiretroviral therapy is currently recommended to consist of two antiretrovirals and possibly a protease inhibitor, with monotherapy with ZDV being suboptimal. There is limited experience with the use of other antiretrovirals, such as lamivudine, stavudine, and protease inhibitors, during pregnancy, despite the theoretical risk to the fetus from combination therapy. Some people have suggested stopping these treatments during the first trimester and starting combinations again, but doing so also carries the risk of resistance developing. Any antiretroviral medication should be given to the women with an explanation of the available knowledge and a recommendation for long-term child monitoring.

Care During Labour and Delivery

Most of the time, HIV-positive women should receive routine labor and delivery care. As mother-to-child transmission increases when membranes are ruptured for more than four hours, prolonged membrane rupture should be avoided.If labor progress is sufficient, membranes should not be artificially ruptured. This could be made a standard part of labor management for all women in high-prevalence areas due to its benefits.Due to the unconfirmed magnitude of the risk for HIV transmission, any procedure that breaks the baby's skin or increases the baby's contact with the mother's blood, such as scalp electrodes or scalp blood sampling, should be avoided unless absolutely necessary. When managing pregnant women, universal precautions should be taken in all instances. Episiotomy should only be performed in obstetrical cases and should not be performed on a regular basis. Due to the possibility of scalp micro-lacerations from the vacuum cup, forceps may be preferable to vacuum extraction if assisted delivery is required. There is more and more evidence to suggest that elective cesarean sections may aid in preventing HIV transmission to the unborn child.In

HIV-positive women, the procedure is associated with an increased risk of maternal complications and post-operative morbidity. Each person should make their own decision about whether or not to have a cesarean section. Both elective and emergency cesarean sections should be treated with preventative antibiotics.

Postpartum Care

HIV-positive women should receive the same postpartum care as healthy women. They don't need their own nursing homes. However, if women decide not to breastfeed in a culture that is likely to condemn such behavior, they may need private facilities to lessen the social stigma associated with it. Postpartum infectious complications, such as wound infections in the urinary tract, chest, episiotomy, and cesarean section, are more common in HIV-positive women.Health care providers ought to be aware of this and keep an eye out for signs of infection. When there is a short postpartum hospital stay, mothers should be informed about the early signs of infection at discharge. All mothers should be taught how to properly care for their perineum and how to handle lochia and blood-stained sanitary products or materials. Information on how to care for babies without putting them at risk of infection and a thorough discussion of the dangers and benefits of feeding infants should be provided to mothers . If the mother is not breastfeeding, she should be given all the information she needs to know about safe formula feeding, and lactation should be discouraged. When a child has cracked nipples, mastitis, a breast abscess, or oral lesions, mothers who choose to breastfeed should be informed of the increased transmission risk. If it is safe to do so, it may be encouraged to shorten the duration of breastfeeding and encourage early weaning. The mother should be advised about the options for child testing and the need for follow-up care for her and her child.She ought to be informed about and referred to HIV support groups in her area. In order to begin with the appropriate method, contraceptive advice should be given and early arrangements should be made.

Care of Neonates

Babies born to mothers who are HIV positive should be handled with gloves until the mother's blood and secretions are washed away, at which point they can be handled safely by both the mother and the health care provider. When the child received six weeks of long-term treatment with ZDV, the most common complication was anemia. If this regimen is followed, hemoglobin levels should be measured at the beginning, six weeks, and twelve weeks. The risk of anemia is significantly lower with short-course therapies. Hepatic transaminases may temporarily rise in infants receiving long-term antiretrovirals. More intensive hematological monitoring would be recommended because there is less experience with the use of combination therapy in pregnant women and the risk of toxicity to these infants. Before giving birth, mothers should choose how to feed their children and should be supported in doing so. Children should be referred for long-term follow-up and repeat HIV testing, either using ELISA at 15 to 18 months or early PCR if available.